Slow Cooker Tasty Recipes

Enjoy These Delicious recipes for everyday Meals

Donna Conway

Table of Contents

5

Artichoke Spinach Dip

Preparation time: 10 minutes

Cooking time: 6 hours

Servings: 4 people

Ingredients:

- 8 oz cream cheese, softened

- 14 oz artichoke hearts, chopped

- 10 oz frozen spinach, thawed and drained

- 1/4 tsp garlic powder

- 2 tbsp water

- 2 cups of cottage cheese

- 1 tsp salt

Directions:

1. Add spinach, cream cheese, cottage cheese, water, and artichoke hearts to a slow cooker and stir well. Season with garlic powder and salt. Cover and cook on low within 6 hours. Stir well and serve.

Nutrition:

Calories: 230

Fat: 14.8g

Carbs: 8.9g

Protein: 15.7g

Tomato Dip

Preparation time: 10 minutes

Cooking time: 1 hour

Servings: 4 people

Ingredients:

- 8 oz cream cheese

- 1/4 cup sun-dried tomatoes

- 1 tbsp mayonnaise

- 3 garlic cloves

- 1/4 tsp white pepper

- 1 tsp pine nuts, toasted

- 3/4 oz fresh basil

Directions:

1. Add all fixings to a blender and blend until smooth. Pour mixture into a slow cooker. Cover and cook on low for 1 hour. Stir well and serve.

Nutrition: Calories: 47 Fat: 4.5g Carbs: 1g Protein: 1g

Italian Mushrooms

Preparation time: 10 minutes

Cooking time: 4 hours

Serves: 4 people

Ingredients:

- 1 lb. mushrooms, cleaned

- 1 onion, sliced

- 1 packet Italian dressing mix

- 1/2 cup butter, melted

Directions:

1. Add onion and mushrooms to a slow cooker and mix well. Combine butter and Italian dressing mix and pour over the onion and mushrooms. Cover and cook on low for 4 hours. Serve and enjoy.

Nutrition:

Calories: 162

Fat: 15.6g

Carbs: 4.8g

Protein: 2.8g

Garlic Cheese Spinach

Preparation time: 10 minutes

Cooking time: 1 hour

Servings: 4 people

Ingredients:

- 16 oz baby spinach

- 2 garlic cloves, minced

- 1 cup cheddar cheese, shredded

- 3 oz cream cheese

Directions:

1. Add all fixings to a slow cooker and stir well. Cover and cook on high within 1 hour. Stir well and serve.

Nutrition: Calories: 216 Fat: 17.2g Carbs: 5.6g Protein: 12g

Dill Carrots

Preparation time: 10 minutes

Cooking time: 2 hours

Serving: 4 people

Ingredients:

- 1 lb. carrots, peeled and cut into round pieces on the diagonal

- 1 tbsp butter

- 1 tbsp fresh dill, minced

- 3 tbsp water

Directions:

1. Add all fixings to a slow cooker and stir well. Cover and cook on low for 2 hours. Stir well and serve.

Nutrition:

Calories: 49

Fat: 1.9g

Carbs: 7.7g

Protein: 0.7g

Rosemary Green Beans

Preparation time: 10 minutes

Cooking time: 1 hour 30 minutes

Servings: 4 people

Ingredients:

- 1 lb. green beans, washed and trimmed

- 2 tbsp fresh lemon juice

- 1 tsp fresh thyme, minced

- 2 tbsp water

- 1 tbsp fresh rosemary, minced

Directions:

1. Add all fixings to a slow cooker and stir well. Cover and cook on low for 1 hour and 30 minutes. Stir well and serve.

Nutrition:

Calories: 40

Fat: 0.4g

Carbs: 8.9g

Protein: 2.2g

Vegetable Fajitas

Preparation time: 10 minutes

Cooking time: 3 hours 30 minutes

Servings: 4 people

Ingredients:

- 1 cup cherry tomatoes, halved

- 3 bell peppers, cut into strips

- 1 onion, sliced

- 1 tsp paprika

- 1 tbsp olive oil

- Pepper and salt

Directions:

1. Add onion, bell peppers, oil, smoked paprika, pepper, and salt to a slow cooker and stir well. Cover and cook on high within 1 hour and 30 minutes. Add cherry tomatoes and cook for 2 hours longer. Stir well and serve.

Nutrition:

Calories: 79

Fat: 3.9g

Carbs: 11.4g

Protein: 1.7g

Roasted Broccoli

Preparation time: 10 minutes

Cooking time: 2 hours

Servings: 4 people

Ingredients:

- 2 lb. broccoli florets

- 1 bell pepper, chopped

- 2 tsp olive oil

- Pepper and salt

Directions:

1. Add all fixings to a slow cooker and stir well to mix. Cover and cook on high for 2 hours. Stir well and serve.

Nutrition:

Calories: 89

Fat: 3.2g

Carbs: 13.3g

Protein: 7g

Tomatoes, Garlic and Okra

Preparation time: 10 minutes

Cooking time: 2 hours

Servings: 4 people

Ingredients:

- 1 1/2 cups okra, diced

- 1 small onion, diced

- 2 large tomatoes, diced

- 1 tsp hot sauce

- 2 garlic cloves, minced

Directions:

1. Add all fixings to a slow cooker and stir well. Cover and cook on low for 2 hours. Stir well and serve.

Nutrition:

Calories: 41

Fat: 0.3g

Carbs: 8.5g

Protein: 1.8g

Cauliflower Rice

Preparation time: 10 minutes

Cooking time: 2 hours

Servings: 4 people

Ingredients:

- 4 cups cauliflower, shredded

- 1 cup vegetable stock

- 1 cup of water

- 1 tablespoon cream cheese

- 1 teaspoon dried oregano

Directions:

1. Put all ingredients in the slow cooker. Close the lid and cook the cauliflower rice on high for 2 hours. Serve.

Nutrition:

Calories: 25

Protein: 0.8g

Carbs: 3.9g

Fat: 0.8g

Squash Noodles

Preparation time: 15 minutes

Cooking time: 4 hours

Servings: 4 people

Ingredients:

- 1-pound butternut squash, seeded, halved

- 1 tablespoon vegan butter

- 1 teaspoon salt

- ½ teaspoon garlic powder

- 3 cups of water

Directions:

1. Pour water into the slow cooker. Add butternut squash and close the lid. Cook the vegetable on high for 4 hours.

2. Then drain water and shred the squash flesh with the fork's help and transfer in the bowl. Add garlic powder, salt, and butter. Mix the squash noodles.

Nutrition:

Calories: 78

Protein: 1.2g

Carbs: 13.5g

Fat: 3g

Thyme Tomatoes

Preparation time: 15 minutes

Cooking time: 5 hours

Servings: 4 people

Ingredients:

- 1-pound tomatoes, sliced

- 1 tablespoon dried thyme

- 1 teaspoon salt

- 2 tablespoons olive oil

- 1 tablespoon apple cider vinegar

- ½ cup of water

Directions:

1. Put all fixings in the slow cooker and close the lid. Cook the tomatoes on low for 5 hours. Serve.

Nutrition:

Calories: 83

Protein: 1.1g

Carbs: 4.9g

Fat: 7.3g

Quinoa Dolma

Preparation time: 15 minutes

Cooking time: 4 hours

Servings: 4 people

Ingredients:

- 6 sweet peppers, seeded

- 1 cup quinoa, cooked

- ½ cup corn kernels, cooked

- 1 teaspoon chili flakes

- 1 cup of water

- ½ cup tomato juice

Directions:

1. Mix quinoa with corn kernels and chili flakes. Fill the

   sweet peppers with quinoa mixture and put them in

the slow cooker. Add water and tomato juice. Close the lid and cook the peppers on high for 3 hours. Serve.

Nutrition:

Calories: 171

Protein: 6.6g

Carbs: 33.7g

Fat: 2.3g

Creamy Puree

Preparation time: 15 minutes

Cooking time: 4 hours

Servings: 4 people

Ingredients:

- 2 cups potatoes, chopped

- 3 cups of water

- 1 tablespoon vegan butter

- ¼ cup cream

- 1 teaspoon salt

Directions:

1. Pour water into the slow cooker. Add potatoes and

   salt. Cook the vegetables on high for 4 hours. Then

drain water, add butter and cream. Mash the potatoes until smooth. Serve.

Nutrition:

Calories: 87

Protein: 1.4g

Carbs: 12.3g

Fat: 3.8g

Cauliflower Hash

Preparation time: 15 minutes

Cooking time: 2 hours & 30 minutes

Servings: 4 people

Ingredients:

- 3 cups cauliflower, roughly chopped

- ½ cup potato, chopped

- 3 oz Provolone, grated

- 2 tablespoons chives, chopped

- 1 cup milk

- ½ cup of water

- 1 teaspoon chili powder

Directions:

1. Pour water and milk into the slow cooker. Add cauliflower, potato, chives, and chili powder. Close the lid and cook the mixture on high for 2 hours. Then sprinkle the hash with provolone cheese and cook the meal on high for 30 minutes.

Nutrition:

Calories: 134

Protein: 9.3g

Carbs: 9.5g

Fat: 7.1g

Cheesy Corn

Preparation time: 5 minutes

Cooking time: 5 hours

Servings: 4 people

Ingredients:

- 4 cups corn kernels

- ½ cup Cheddar cheese, shredded

- 1 tablespoon vegan butter

- 1 teaspoon ground black pepper

- 1 teaspoon salt

- 2 cups of water

Directions:

1. Mix corn kernels with ground black pepper, butter, salt, and cheese. Transfer the batter to your slow

cooker and add water. Close the lid and cook the meal on low for 5 hours. Serve.

Nutrition:

Calories: 173

Protein: 6.9g

Carbs: 23.6g

Fat: 7.5g

Shredded Cabbage Sauté

Preparation time: 10 minutes

Cooking time: 6 hours

Servings: 4 people

Ingredients:

- 3 cups white cabbage, shredded

- 1 cup tomato juice

- 1 teaspoon salt

- 1 teaspoon sugar

- 1 teaspoon dried oregano

- 3 tablespoons olive oil

- 1 cup of water

Directions:

1. Put all ingredients in the slow cooker. Carefully mix all ingredients with the help of the spoon and close the lid. Cook the cabbage sauté for 6 hours on low. Serve.

Nutrition:

Calories: 118

Protein: 1.2g

Carbs: 6.9g

Fat: 10.6g

Ranch Broccoli

Preparation time: 15 minutes

Cooking time: 1 hour & 30 minutes

Servings: 3 people

Ingredients:

- 3 cups broccoli

- 1 teaspoon chili flakes

- 2 tablespoons ranch dressing

- 2 cups of water

Directions:

1. Put the broccoli in the slow cooker. Add water and close the lid. Cook the broccoli on high for 1 hour and 30 minutes.

2. Then drain water and transfer the broccoli to the bowl. Sprinkle it with chili flakes and ranch dressing. Shake the meal gently.

Nutrition:

Calories: 34

Protein: 2.7g

Carbs: 6.6g

Fat: 0.3g

Cheddar Mushrooms

Preparation time: 10 minutes

Cooking time: 6 hours

Servings: 4 people

Ingredients:

- 4 cups cremini mushrooms, sliced

- 1 teaspoon dried oregano

- 1 teaspoon ground black pepper

- ½ teaspoon salt

- 1 cup Cheddar cheese, shredded

- 1 cup heavy cream

- 1 cup of water

Directions:

1. Pour water and heavy cream into the slow cooker. Add salt, ground black pepper, and dried oregano. Then add sliced mushrooms and cheddar cheese.

2. Cook the meal on low for 6 hours. When the mushrooms are cooked, gently stir them and transfer them to the serving plates.

Nutrition:

Calories: 239

Protein: 9.6g

Carbs: 4.8g

Fat: 20.6g

Paprika Baby Carrot

Preparation time: 10 minutes

Cooking time: 2 hours & 30 minutes

Servings: 2 people

Ingredients:

- 1 tablespoon ground paprika

- 2 cups baby carrot

- 1 teaspoon cumin seeds

- 1 cup of water

- 1 teaspoon vegan butter

Directions:

1. Pour water into the slow cooker. Add baby carrot, cumin seeds, and ground paprika. Close the lid and

cook the carrot on high for 2 hours and 30 minutes. Then drain water, add butter, and shake the vegetables. Serve.

Nutrition:

Calories: 60

Protein: 1.6g

Carbs: 8.6g

Fat: 2.7g

Butter Asparagus

Preparation time: 15 minutes

Cooking time: 5 hours

Servings: 4 people

Ingredients:

- 1-pound asparagus

- 2 tablespoons vegan butter

- 1 teaspoon ground black pepper

- 1 cup vegetable stock

Directions:

1. Pour the vegetable stock into the slow cooker. Chop the asparagus roughly and add to the slow cooker.

Close the lid and cook the asparagus for 5 hours on low.

2. Then drain water and transfer the asparagus to the bowl. Sprinkle it with ground black pepper and butter.

Nutrition:

Calories: 77

Protein: 2.8g

Carbs: 4.9g

Fat: 6.1g

Jalapeno Corn

Preparation time: 10 minutes

Cooking time: 5 hours

Servings: 4 people

Ingredients:

- 1 cup heavy cream

- ½ cup Monterey Jack cheese, shredded

- 1-pound corn kernels

- 3 jalapenos, minced

- 1 teaspoon vegan butter

- 1 tablespoon dried dill

Directions:

1. Pour heavy cream into the slow cooker. Add

   Monterey Jack cheese, corn kernels, minced

jalapeno, butter, and dried dill. Cook the corn on low for 5 hours. Serve.

Nutrition:

Calories: 203

Protein: 5.6g

Carbs: 9.3g

Fat: 16.9g

Mashed Turnips

Preparation time: 10 minutes

Cooking time: 7 hours

Servings: 4 people

Ingredients:

- 3-pounds turnip, chopped

- 3 cups of water

- 1 tablespoon vegan butter

- 1 tablespoon chives, chopped

- 2 oz Parmesan, grated

Directions:

1. Put turnips in the slow cooker. Add water and cook the vegetables on low for 7 hours. Then drain water and mash the turnips.

2. Add chives, butter, and parmesan. Carefully stir the mixture until butter and parmesan are melted. Then add chives. Remix the mashed turnips.

Nutrition:

Calories: 162

Protein: 8.6g

Carbs: 15.1g

Fat: 8.1g

Cranberry, Apple, and Squash Dish

Preparation time: 15 minutes

Cooking time: 4 hours

Servings: 2 people

Ingredients:

- ¾ pound butternut squash, cubed and peeled

- 1 apple, cored, peeled, and chopped

- 2 tbsp. cranberries, dried

- ¼ diced onion

- ½ tsp. cinnamon

- ¼ tsp. nutmeg

Directions:

1. First, add the squash, apple, cranberries, onion, cinnamon, and nutmeg to the slow cooker. Stir well. Cook on high within 4 hours. Stir well, and serve warm.

Nutrition:

Calories: 72

Carbs: 17g

Fat: 0g

Protein: 0g

Vegetarian Curry with Indian Spices

Preparation time: 15 minutes

Cooking time: 5 hours

Servings: 4 people

Ingredients:

- 2 potatoes, cubed

- 2 tbsp curry powder

- ½ red pepper, sliced

- 1 tbsp flour

- ½ ounce dried onion soup mix

- 1 tsp chili powder

- ¼ tsp red pepper flakes

- ¼ tsp cayenne pepper

- ½ sliced green pepper

- 7 oz. coconut cream, unsweetened

- 1 cup sliced carrots

- 2 tbsp fresh cilantro, chopped, for garnish

Directions:

1. Add the potatoes to the slow cooker. Stir together the flour, curry powder, chili powder, red pepper flakes, and cayenne pepper in a medium-sized bowl. Sprinkle this spice mixture over the potatoes. Stir well.

2. Add the peppers, onion soup mix, and coconut cream to the slow cooker. Stir well. Cover the slow cooker. Cook the mixture on low within 4 hours. As the mixture cooks, add water to keep the mix moist.

3. Add the carrots to the mixture—Cook for an additional 60 minutes. Add the cilantro for garnish, and serve the meal warm.

Nutrition:

Calories: 300

Carbs: 36g

Fat: 6g

Protein: 21g

Parsnip, Turnip, and Carrot Tagine

Preparation time: 15 minutes

Cooking time: 9 hours

Servings: 4 people

Ingredients:

- ½ pound peeled and diced parsnips

- 1 diced onion

- ½ pound peeled and diced turnips

- ½ pound diced and peeled carrots

- 3 chopped apricots, dried

- ½ tsp. turmeric

- 2 chopped prunes

- ¼ tsp. ginger

- ¼ tsp. cinnamon

- 1 tsp. dried parsley

- 1 tsp. dried cilantro

- 7 oz. vegetable broth

Directions:

1. Add the parsnips, onion, turnips, carrots, apricots, turmeric, prunes, ginger, cinnamon, parsley, cilantro, and the broth to the slow cooker. Cook the mixture on low for 9 hours. Serve warm, and enjoy.

Nutrition: Calories: 246 Carbs: 8g Fat: 2g Protein: 1g

Spinach and Pumpkin Chili

Preparation time: 15 minutes

Cooking time: 4 hours & 30 minutes

Servings: 4 people

Ingredients:

- 14 oz. diced tomatoes

- 7 oz. pure pumpkin puree

- 1/3 cup vegetable juice

- 1/3 cup chopped okra

- 1/3 cup chopped broccoli

- 1 tbsp. sugar

- ½ diced zucchini

- ½ diced onion

- 2 tsp. pumpkin pie spice

- ½ tsp. chili powder

- ½ tsp. salt

- 9 oz. fava beans

- 1 cup chopped spinach

- 2 tsp. white vinegar

Directions:

1. Add the tomatoes, pumpkin, okra, vegetable juice, sugar, broccoli, carrot, zucchini, onion, pumpkin pie spice, vinegar, chili powder, pepper, and salt the slow cooker.

2. Cook the chili on high within 4 hours. Stir in the spinach and the fava beans. Cook for another 30 minutes on high. Serve warm, and enjoy.

Nutrition: Calories: 125 Carbs: 16g Fat: 6g Protein: 2g

Veggie-Friendly Buffalo Dip

Preparation time: 15 minutes

Cooking time: 2 hours

Servings: 4 people

Ingredients:

- 8 oz. chicken-style vegetarian strips, diced

- 16 oz. low-fat ranch salad dressing

- 16 oz. cream cheese, softened

- 12 oz. hot sauce

- 1 cup Colby Jack cheese, shredded

Directions:

1. Add the fake chicken strips, cream cheese, hot sauce, and ranch dressing to the slow cooker. Stir well, and heat on low for 2 hours. Add the shredded cheese to the mixture. Stir well, and serve warm.

Nutrition:

Calories: 60

Carbs: 2g

Fat: 5g

Protein: 1g

Split Black Lentils with Curry

Preparation time: 15 minutes

Cooking time: 5 hours

Servings: 4 people

Ingredients:

- 3 cups of water

- 1 cup split black lentils

- 1 minced garlic clove

- ¼ chopped onion

- 1 tsp. sugar

- ½ tsp. turmeric powder

- 1 tsp. curry powder

- 1/3 cup heavy cream

- ½ inch of fresh ginger

- Salt to taste

Directions:

1. Add the water, onion, lentils, garlic, salt, sugar, curry powder, ginger root, and turmeric to the slow cooker. Stir well.

2. Cook on high within 5 hours. Put the cream in the slow cooker, stir until well combined, and serve warm.

Nutrition:

Calories: 275

Carbs: 41g

Fat: 1g

Protein: 25g

Mulled Wine

Preparation time: 5 minutes

Cooking time: 2 hours

Servings: 8 glasses

Ingredients:

- 6 cups sweet red wine

- 1 cup apple cider

- 1/4 cup light brown sugar

- 1 small orange, sliced

- 1 cinnamon stick

- 4 whole cloves

- 2-star anise

- 4 cardamom pods, crushed

Directions:

1. Combine all the fixings in your slow cooker. Cover the pot and cook for 2 hours on high. The mulled wine is best served warm.

Nutrition:

Calories: 227

Carbs: 29g

Fat: 0g

Protein: 0g

Cranberry Spiced Tea

Preparation time: 5 minutes

Cooking time: 2 hours

Servings: 6 glasses

Ingredients:

- 4 cups of water
- 1 cup strong brewed black tea
- 1 cup cranberry juice
- 1/2 cup white sugar
- 2 cinnamon stick
- 2-star anise
- 2 cardamom pods, crushed
- 1 lemon, sliced

Directions:

1. Combine all the fixings in your slow cooker. Cook on high settings for 2 hours. Serve the drink warm.

Nutrition: Calories: 80 Carbs: 22g Fat: 0g Protein: 0g

Rosemary Mulled Cider

Preparation time: 15 minutes

Cooking time: 3 hours

Servings: 6 glasses

Ingredients:

- 4 cups apple cider

- 2 cups rose wine

- 1 cup fresh or frozen cranberries

- 1 rosemary sprig

- 1/2 cup white sugar

- 1 cinnamon stick

- 2 whole cloves

Directions:

1. Combine all the fixings in your slow cooker. Cover and cook for 3 hours on low settings. Serve the beverage warm.

Nutrition: Calories: 165 Carbs: 43g Fat: 0g n Protein: 0g

Gingerbread Hot Chocolate

Preparation time: 15 minutes

Cooking time: 2 hours

Servings: 8 glasses

Ingredients:

- 6 cups whole milk

- 1 cup dark chocolate chips

- 1 cup sweetened condensed milk

- 2 tablespoons cocoa powder

- 1/2 teaspoon ground ginger

- 2 cinnamon stick

- 2 tablespoons maple syrup

- 1 pinch salt

Directions:

1. Combine all the fixings in your slow cooker. Cover the pot and cook for 2 hours on high settings. Serve the hot chocolate warm.

Nutrition:

Calories: 140

Carbs: 29g

Fat: 3g

Protein: 2g

Gingerbread Mocha Drink

Preparation time: 5 minutes

Cooking time: 1 hour & 30 minutes

Servings: 6 glasses

Ingredients:

- 3 cups whole milk

- 2 cups strongly brewed coffee

- 1/2 cup sweetened condensed milk

- 1/4 cup light brown sugar

- 1/2 teaspoon ground ginger

- 1/4 teaspoon cinnamon powder

- 1/4 teaspoon cardamom powder

Directions:

1. Combine all the fixings in a slow cooker. Cover the pot and cook for 1 1/2 hours on low settings. Serve the mocha drink warm.

Nutrition: Calories: 270 Carbs: 40g Fat: 7g Protein: 12g

Salted Caramel Milk Steamer

Preparation time: 15 minutes

Cooking time: 2 hours

Servings: 6 glasses

Ingredients:

- 4 cups whole milk
- 1 cup heavy cream
- 1 cup caramel sauce
- 1/4 teaspoon salt
- 1/4 teaspoon ground ginger
- 1 teaspoon vanilla extract

Directions:

1. Combine all the fixings in your slow cooker. Cook within 2 hours on low. Pour the steamer into glasses or mugs and serve right away.

Nutrition: Calories: 150 Carbs: 28g Fat: 0g Protein: 10g

Apple Chai Tea

Preparation time: 15 minutes

Cooking time: 4 hours

Servings: 8 glasses

Ingredients:

- 4 cups brewed black tea
- 4 cups fresh apple juice
- 1/3 cup white sugar
- 2 red apples, cored and diced
- 2 cinnamon stick
- 1-star anise
- 2 whole cloves
- 2 cardamom pods, crushed

Directions:

1. Combine all the fixings in your slow cooker. Cook the tea on low settings for 4 hours. Serve the tea warm.

Nutrition: Calories: 170 Carbs: 0g Fat: 0g Protein: 0

Ginger Pumpkin Latte

Preparation time: 15 minutes

Cooking time: 3 hours

Servings: 6 glasses

Ingredients:

- 4 cups whole milk
- 1 cup pumpkin puree
- 1 cup brewed coffee
- 1/4 cup dark brown sugar
- 1 teaspoon ground ginger
- 1 cinnamon stick
- 1 pinch nutmeg

Directions:

1. Combine all the fixings in a slow cooker. Cover the pot and cook for 3 hours on low settings. Serve the latte warm.

Nutrition: Calories: 422 Carbs: 57g Fat: 17g Protein: 10g

Hot Caramel Apple Drink

Preparation time: 15 minutes

Cooking time: 2 hours

Servings: 8 glasses

Ingredients:

- 6 cups apple cider

- 1 cup apple liqueur

- 1 cup light rum

- 1/2 cup caramel syrup

- 2 red apples, cored and diced

- 2 cinnamon stick

Directions:

1. Mix all the ingredients in your slow cooker. Cover the pot and cook for 2 hours on low settings.

Nutrition: Calories: 116 Carbs: 29g Fat: 0g Protein: 0g

Spiced White Chocolate

Preparation time: 15 minutes

Cooking time: 1 hour & 30 minutes

Servings: 6 glasses

Ingredients:

- 4 cups whole milk

- 1 cup sweetened condensed milk

- 1 cup white chocolate chips

- 1 cinnamon stick

- 1-star anise

- 1/2-inch piece of ginger, sliced

- 1 pinch nutmeg

Directions:

1. Combine all the fixings in your slow cooker. Cover it and cook for 1 1/2 hours on low settings. Serve the drink hot.

Nutrition: Calories: 430 Carbs: 42g Fat: 24g Protein: 11g

Apple Bourbon Punch

Preparation time: 15 minutes

Cooking time: 2 hours

Servings: 4 glasses

Ingredients:

- 3 cups apple cider
- 1 cup bourbon
- 1/2 cup fresh or frozen cranberries
- 2 cinnamon stick
- 2 whole cloves
- 1/4 cup light brown sugar

Directions:

1. Combine all the fixings in your slow cooker and cook for 2 hours on low settings. Serve the drink hot.

Nutrition: Calories: 60 Carbs: 2g Fat: 0g Protein: 0g

Maple Bourbon Mulled Cider

Preparation time: 15 minutes

Cooking time: 1 hour & 30 minutes

Servings: 6 glasses

Ingredients:

- 5 cups apple cider
- 1/2 cup bourbon
- 1/2 cup fresh apple juice
- 1/4 cup maple syrup
- 2-star anise

Directions:

1. Mix all the ingredients in your slow cooker. Cover the pot and cook for 1 1/2 hours on low settings. Serve hot.

Nutrition: Calories: 120 Carbs: 28g Fat: 0g Protein: 0g

Autumn Punch

Preparation time: 15 minutes

Cooking time: 4 hours

Servings: 8 glasses

Ingredients:

- 6 cups red wine

- 1 cup bourbon

- 1 cup cranberry juice

- 1 vanilla bean, split in half lengthwise

- 2 red apples, cored and diced

- 1 ripe pear, cored and sliced

- 1 cinnamon stick

- 2 whole cloves

Directions:

1. Combine all the fixings in your slow cooker. Cover and cook within 4 hours on low settings. The punch can be served both hot and chilled.

Nutrition:

Calories: 140

Carbs: 37g

Fat: 0g

Protein: 0g

Hot Spicy Apple Cider

Preparation time: 15 minutes

Cooking time: 3 hours

Servings: 6 glasses

Ingredients:

- 5 cups apple cider
- 1 cup white rum
- 2 cinnamon stick
- 1/4 teaspoon chili powder
- 1-star anise
- 1 orange, sliced

Directions:

1. Combine all the fixings in your slow cooker. Cover the pot and cook for 3 hours on low settings. Serve the cider warm.

Nutrition: Calories: 60 Carbs: 15g Fat: 0g Protein: 0g

Vanilla Latte

Preparation time: 15 minutes

Cooking time: 2 hours

Servings: 6 glasses

Ingredients:

- 4 cups whole milk

- 2 cups brewed coffee

- 1 vanilla pod, split in half lengthwise

- 1/4 cup sweetened condensed milk

Directions:

1. Combine all the fixings in your slow cooker. Cover and cook for 2 hours on low settings. Serve the latte warm.

Nutrition: Calories: 73 Carbs: 13g Fat: 2g Protein: 2g

Chicken and Rice Stew

Preparation time: 15 minutes

Cooking time: 8 hours

Servings: 4 people

Ingredients:

- 2 medium carrots
- 2 medium leeks
- 1 cup rice, uncooked
- 12 oz boneless chicken, without skin
- 1 tsp. thyme
- ½ tsp. rosemary
- 3 cans of chicken broth
- 1 can cream of mushroom soup
- ½ cup onion, chopped
- 1 clove garlic

Directions:

1. Place all the fixings in a slow cooker. Cover the slow cooker. Cook on low for 7 or 8 hours. or on high for 4 hours. Serve hot.

Nutrition:

Calories: 245.5

Fat: 6.2g

Carbs: 21.2g

Protein: 25.2g

Chicken and Tortilla Soup

Preparation time: 15 minutes

Cooking time: 6-8 hours

Servings: 4 people

Ingredients:

- 3 chicken breasts, boneless and skinless

- 15 oz. diced tomatoes

- 10 oz. enchilada sauce

- 1 chopped onion, medium

- 4 oz. chopped chili pepper, green

- 3 minced cloves garlic

- 2 cups of water

- 14.5-oz. chicken broth, fat-free

- 1 tbsp. cumin

- 1 tbs. chili powder

- 1 tsp. salt

- ¼ tsp. black pepper

- bay leaf

- 1 tbsp. cilantro, chopped

- 10 oz. of frozen corn

- 3 tortillas, cut into thin slices

Directions:

1. Place all the ingredients in the slow cooker. Stir well to mix. Cook on low heat for 8 hours or on high heat for 6 hours.

2. Transfer the chicken breasts to a plate and shred. Add chicken to other ingredients. Serve hot, garnished with tortilla slices.

Nutrition:

Calories: 93.4

Fat: 1.9g

Carbs: 11.9g

Protein: 8.3g

Stuffed Pepper Soup

Preparation time: 15 minutes

Cooking time: 8 hours

Servings: 4 people

Ingredients:

- 1 lb. ground beef, drained

- 1 chopped onion, large

- 2 cups tomatoes, diced

- 2 chopped green peppers

- 2 cups tomato sauce

- 1 tbsp beef bouillon

- 3 cups of water

- pepper

- 1 tsp. of salt

- 1 cup of cooked rice, white

Directions:

1. Place all fixings in a slow cooker. Cook for 8 hours on low. Serve hot.

Nutrition:

Calories: 216.1

Fat: 5.1g

Carbs: 21.8mg

Protein: 18.8g

Ham and Pea Soup

Preparation time: 15 minutes

Cooking time: 8 hours

Servings: 4 people

Ingredients:

- 1 lb. split peas, dried
- 1 cup sliced celery
- 1 cup sliced carrots
- 1 cup sliced onion
- 2 cups chopped ham, cooked
- 8 cups of water

Directions:

1. Place all the ingredients in the slow cooker. Cook on low for 8 hours. Serve hot.

Nutrition: Calories: 118.6 Fat: 1.9g Carbs: 14.5mg Protein: 11.1g

Vegetable Stew

Preparation time: 15 minutes

Cooking time: 8 hours

Servings: 4 people

Ingredients:

- 1 cup of corn

- 1 cup hominy

- 1 cup green beans

- 1 can peas, black-eyed

- 1 cup lima beans

- 1 cup chopped carrots

- 1 cup chopped celery

- 1 cup onion

- 1 can tomato sauce, small

- 2 cups vegetable broth

- 2 tbsp. Worcestershire sauce

Directions:

1. Place all the ingredients in the slow cooker. Cook on low for 8 hours. Serve hot.

Nutrition:

Calories: 186

Fat: 1.2g

Carbs: 38.8mg

Protein: 8.3g

Pea Soup

Preparation time: 15 minutes

Cooking time: 8 hours

Servings: 4 people

Ingredients:

- 16 oz. split peas, dried

- 1 cup chopped baby carrots

- 1chopped onion, white

- 3 bay leaves

- 10 oz. cubed turkey ham

- 4 cubes chicken bouillon

- 7 cups of water

Directions:

1. Rinse and drain peas. Place all the ingredients in the slow cooker. Cook on low for 8 hrs. Serve hot.

Nutrition:

Calories: 122.7

Fat: 2g

Carbs: 15mg

Protein: 11.8g

Soup for The Day

Preparation time: 15 minutes

Cooking time: 10 hours

Servings: 4 people

Ingredients:

- 1 beefsteak, cubed

- 1 chopped onion, medium

- 1 tbsp. olive oil

- 5 thinly sliced medium carrots

- 4 cups cabbage

- 4 diced red potatoes

- 2 diced celery stalks

- 2 cans tomatoes, diced

- 2 cans beef broth

- 1 tsp. sugar

- 1 can tomato soup

- 1 tsp. parsley flakes, dried

- 2 tsp. Italian seasoning

Directions:

1. In a skillet, sauté onion and steak in oil. Transfer the sautéed mixture to the slow cooker. Put the rest of the fixings in the slow cooker. Cook on low for 10 hours. Serve hot.

Nutrition:

Calories: 259.6

Fat: 6.7g

Carbs: 31.6mg

Protein: 18.9g

Pork and Fennel Stew

Preparation time: 15 minutes

Cooking time: 8 hours & 10 minutes

Servings: 4 people

Ingredients:

- 8 cups of fennel, thinly sliced

- 1 onion, halved and sliced

- 2 ½ pounds pork shoulder, cubed

- 1 ½ tsp. kosher salt

- 1 ½ tsp. pepper, grounded

- 2 tbsp. olive oil, extra virgin

- ¾ cup white wine, dry

- 4 cloves minced garlic

- 1 tbsp. chopped rosemary

- 2 tsp. chopped oregano

- 28 ounce can tomato, whole

Directions:

1. Place onion and fennel on the bottom of the slow cooker. In another dish, sprinkle the pepper and salt on pork. In a skillet, pour in the oil.

2. Brown the pork that will fit in the skillet for 5 minutes. Transfer the pork to the slow cooker.

3. Put the wine into the pan, then scrape the brown pieces in the pan. Add the rest of the ingredients to the slow cooker. Cook on low for 8 hours. Serve hot.

Nutrition: Calories: 249 Fat: 13g Carbs: 9mg Protein: 20g

Vegetable Garbanzo Stew

Preparation time: 15 minutes

Cooking time: 6 hours & 10 minutes

Servings: 2 people

Ingredients:

- 3 cups diced butternut squash

- 3 peeled and diced carrots

- 2 chopped onions

- 3 minced cloves of garlic

- 4 cups vegetable stock, low sodium

- 1 cup red lentils

- 2 tbsp. tomato paste, unsalted

- 2 tbsp. minced ginger

- 2 tsp. cumin, ground

- 1 tsp. turmeric

- ¼ tsp. saffron

- 1 tsp. pepper, ground

- ¼ cup lemon juice

- 16 oz. garbanzo beans

- ½ cup chopped peanuts, unsalted

- ½ cup chopped cilantro

Directions:

1. Sweat the vegetables in a Dutch oven. Brown the onion. Pour in the stock and scrape any pieces of vegetables sticking to the pan.

2. Now, add all the ingredients to the slow cooker. Cook on low for 6 hours. Stir the lemon juice into the slow cooker before serving. Garnish with peanuts and serve.

Nutrition: Calories: 287 Fat: 8g Carbs: 41mg Protein: 13g

Catalan Stew

Preparation time: 15 minutes

Cooking time: 8 hours & 13 minutes

Servings: 4 people

Ingredients:

- 2 chopped slices of pancetta

- 2 tbsp. olive oil, extra virgin

- 3 pounds chuck roast

- 1 cup red wine, dry

- 2 chopped onions

- 3 cups beef broth, low sodium

- 2 tbsp. tomato paste

- 4 minced cloves garlic

- 2 crushed cinnamon sticks

- 4 sprigs thyme

- 3 slices of peeled orange

- 1 ounce chopped dark chocolate

- 3 tbsp. chopped parsley

Directions:

1. Sauté pancetta in oil till crisp. Transfer it to the slow cooker. Using the same pan, sauté the beef. Transfer beef to the slow cooker as well.

2. Now, sauté onion for 3 minutes. Add wine, tomato paste, and vinegar to the sauté pan and stir to mix. Transfer this wine mixture to the slow cooker and sprinkle on the rest of the ingredients except parsley.

3. Cook on low for 8 hours. Stir when done. Add the chocolate and cook on high for 10 minutes. Remove cinnamon, orange peel, and thyme. Serve after garnishing with parsley.

Nutrition: Calories: 421 Fat: 26g Carbs: 16mg Protein: 55g

Pork Stew Caribbean Style

Preparation time: 15 minutes

Cooking time: 7 hours

Servings: 4 people

Ingredients:

- 1 ½ pounds cubed pork loin

- 1 tbsp. thyme, dried

- ¼ tsp. allspice, ground

- white pepper, ground

- 1-pound Yukon potatoes, quartered

- 3 diced carrots

- 1-inch piece of ginger root, chopped

- 2 tsp. Worcestershire sauce

- 1 chopped clove garlic

- ½ cup sliced scallions

- 1 cup diced tomatoes

Directions:

1. Coat the pork with pepper, allspice, and thyme. Place remaining ingredients except for scallions in the slow cooker. Put in the pork along with the Worcestershire sauce.

2. Place the tomatoes on top. Cook on low for 7 hours. Serve the stew with scallions.

Nutrition: Calories: 452 Fat: 27g Carbs: 25mg Protein: 50g

Kale Verde

Preparation time: 15 minutes

Cooking time: 6 hours

Servings: 4 people

Ingredients:

- ¼ cup olive oil, extra virgin

- 1 yellow onion, large

- 2 cloves garlic

- 2 oz. tomatoes, dried

- 2 cups yellow potatoes, diced

- 14-ounce tomatoes, diced

- 6 cups chicken broth

- white pepper, ground

- 1-pound o chopped kale

Directions:

1. Sauté onion for 5 minutes in oil. Add the garlic and sauté again for 1 minute. Transfer the sautéed mixture to the slow cooker.

2. Now, put the rest of the ingredients except pepper into the slow cooker. Cook on low for 6 hours. Season with white pepper to taste. Serve hot in heated bowls

Nutrition:

Calories: 257

Fat: 22g

Carbs: 27mg

Protein: 14g

Escarole with Bean Soup

Preparation time: 15 minutes

Cooking time: 6 hours

Servings: 4 people

Ingredients:

- 1 tbsp. olive oil

- 8 crushed cloves garlic

- 1 cup chopped onions

- 1 diced carrot

- 3 tsp. basil, dried

- 3 tsp. oregano, dried

- 4 cups chicken broth

- 3 cups chopped escarole

- 1 cup of northern beans, dried

- parmesan cheese, grated

- 14 oz. of tomatoes, diced

Directions:

1. Sauté garlic for 2 minutes in oil using a large soup pot. Except for the cheese, broth, and beans, add the rest of the ingredients and cook for 5 minutes.

2. Transfer the cooked ingredients to the slow cooker. Mix in the broth and beans. Cook on low for 6 hours. Garnish with cheese. Serve hot in heated bowls

Nutrition:

Calories: 98

Fat: 33g

Carbs: 14mg

Protein: 8g

Italian Beef Barley Soup

Preparation time: 10 minutes

Cooking time: 5 hours

Servings: 4 people

Ingredients:

- 2 pounds roasted beef roast

- 5 cups of water

- 4 cubes of beef broth, crumbled

- 1/2 onion, minced

- 1 can of tomato sauce

- 3/4 cup uncooked pearl barley

- salt and pepper to taste

Directions:

1. Combine beef, water, broth, onion, tomato sauce, barley, salt, and pepper in a slow cooker. Cover and cook on low within 5 hours.

Nutrition:

Calories: 512

Fat: 27.8g

Carbs: 35.4g

Protein: 29.7g

www.ingramcontent.com/pod-product-compliance
Lightning Source LLC
Chambersburg PA
CBHW071111030426
42336CB00013BA/2040